HOW I MADE THE RIGHT CHOICE FOR BETTER
HEALTH

CHOICE FOR BETTER
HEALTH

The Whole Food Way to Reverse Disease.

CYNTHIA B. JONES

XULON PRESS

Xulon Press
2301 Lucien Way #415
Maitland, FL 32751
407.339.4217
www.xulonpress.com

Unless otherwise indicated, Scripture quotations taken from the King James Version (KJV)—*public domain.*

Scripture quotations taken from the Amplified Bible (AMP). Copyright © 1954, 1958, 1962, 1964, 1965, 1987 by The Lockman Foundation. Used by permission. All rights reserved.

Scripture quotations taken from the Holy Bible, New International Version (NIV). Copyright © 1973, 1978, 1984, 2011 by Biblica, Inc.™. Used by permission. All rights reserved.

Paperback ISBN-13: 978-1-5456-5431-6
Ebook ISBN-13: 978-1-6305-0597-4

Dedication

This book is dedicated in loving memory of my father, Marvin B. Johnson, who for years battled with sugar diabetes and to my five siblings along with other relatives who have made their departure from this life.

To my mother, Frances Waller for her spiritual wisdom and her love for Holy Spirit.

To my son Ronnell Johnson I dedicate this book also to you son. I give God the praise for your life. Continue to take charge of your health.

Acknowledgements

To my heavenly Father, for His love and grace; for without Him, I would not be able to do anything. Thank You Lord for enabling me to fulfill the purpose of changing and transforming lives by sharing my testimony of your great faithfulness, grace and love.

Xulon Press and Salem Author family, thank you once again for all you've done and for being my book publisher.

Sheree Darien, host of Courageous Conversations, thank you for inviting me to share my story on the "Now Network."

Dr. Tassie Hargrove and Mandy Simmons of Holistic Wellness of Savannah, I appreciate you both so very much for your inspiration and for being a great source of help on my wellness journey.

Sister Judith, thank you for your support my friend and for sharing my testimony to others.

Charles Singleton, my brother in Christ, thank you so much for "the Whole Food Way."

Deanna Whittsett, thank you my dear sister, for the "SWAP."

Ms. Tammie Lee, thank you so very much for your knowledge and skills, "sugar foot."

Pastor Neil and the ODM church family, thank you so very much for your prayers throughout this project.

To the students in the Healing School, thank you for showing up to class, your support, and how together we are making the right choice for better health.

To my son Corey, thank you so much for helping mama through this project and for the "big reveal to come."

To my children, grandchildren, family, church family, and friends I love you so very much from the depths of my heart.

Mema thank you so much "Faith" for your special little prayers for my book. Don't forget yours.

Last but not least, to my dear husband Robert Jones, thank you so much for being my greatest supporter in everything. I love you and appreciate all your patience throughout this project and our wonderful life together sweetie.

Contents

Introduction

It's my greatest passion and purpose to help people live healthy lifestyles and to provide those suffering with sicknesses and debilitating diseases, such as diabetes, high blood pressure, high cholesterol, and obesity, with the necessary tools to reverse disease and to regain optimal health. I strongly believe based on my own experience that through proven lifestyle changes, we can heal our bodies. I decided not to take medical drugs and chose plant-based foods as medication to lower my A1C, cholesterol, and to reverse diabetes and discovered that with proper diet and nutrition, along with daily exercise, that the body can heal itself. It is a fact that some sicknesses and diseases are brought on due to one's heredity, environment, and their ability to handle stress. Some prescription drugs can be helpful in treating the body, however, I believe many of us have been more accustom to thinking of our food as something to enjoy rather than to heal our bodies. We were raised in our homes long ago to eat whatever food that was put on the table, some were good and some were bad. They were foods like chitterlings, pig feet, neck bones, hogshead cheese and so many other poorly nutritious foods. Also as it relates to the healthy side, the good foods were the vegetables we were told to eat before leaving the table, the herbs that grew out in the yard or in the fields. Times have changed from long ago and it seems to be more emphasis put on medicating the body with drugs than with proper nutrition, diet and exercise. Another very important point I want to stress is that I have, and I am sure you too have heard so many people say, "My mother or my father have high blood pressure or diabetes, and that's why I have it too." Or they say, "High blood pressure runs in my family." Well, I hate to be so blunt, but if you want it, you can have it. I don't, and I believe you don't either. So I wrote this book to show you how I fought back and reversed high blood pressure, diabetes, and high cholesterol, and lowered my A1Cs all the natural way. The questions I want to ask you is, are you ready for better health, and are you ready to take your health back? In my book, I will share with you how I:

Said no to the pharmaceutical drug Metformin

Was taken off of high blood pressure medication

Lost forty-eight pounds

Lowered my A1C back to the normal range

Reversed high blood pressure

Reversed diabetes

Lowered my total cholesterol, and more.

You see, I had **high blood pressure**, **high cholesterol**, **diabetes**, **high A1C** and the truth of the matter is if we neglect to take control of our health, some of us will die prematurely, as many already have. With neglect, we will suffer with various diseases in our bodies, have poor quality of health, and be under doctors' care and on pharmaceutical drugs for the rest of our lives. I have made the decision to live and be of good health. In order to live and be of good health, we must take charge of our health. It is our responsibility to eat the right foods and to make it our goal to "eat to live" and not to "live to eat." We all know that some foods are enjoyable to eat, but how often, if at all, do we acknowledge that God created the right foods to keep us healthy and well? I remember this saying from long ago: "You can't get blood from a turnip." Likewise, we cannot expect to be healthy while eating the wrong foods on a continual basis. Are you overweight, obese, or sick? Do you have diabetes, high blood pressure, or high cholesterol, or is your A1C too high? If so, it's time to fight for your health.

It's funny how we can set goals to accomplish many endeavors such as owning a new home, car, business, or planning for the future, etc. But having a healthy lifestyle often doesn't make it to the top of the list. The truth is, investing in our health is far more important because without good health, we cannot enjoy life. So what we eat should be treated with high regard and as an absolute necessity for life.

Well, as I said before, I want to live with the best quality of life and health as I can. There are so many other things to do and places I would like to go, but if my health is poor or failing, nine times out of ten, I will not be able to do those things or go to those places. So my question to you is this, are you ready to take charge of your health and to make the necessary changes in living a healthier life? In my book, I will share with you how I was able to regain my health by making healthy lifestyle choices and if applied you can also receive total recovery of your health.

1. My Wake-Up Call

September 21, 2016, I went to see my primary physician for a routine physical. One of the procedures I had taken was testing of fasting labs, and after having my weight checked, I was in complete shock to find out that I weighed 203.4 pounds, with my blood pressure reading 146/84 and a BMI of 32.83. I was on high blood pressure medication and had been for about thirteen years, yet most times my blood pressure remained elevated. It was during this visit that my eyes were opened and I realized at that particular moment that I had to hit the ground running hard. I knew that this was it for me, I had to lose weight in a hurry. I had become obese and people obesity is dangerous to your health. I will say it again: being obese is dangerous to your health!

I returned on September 28, 2016, one week later, to receive the results of my lab tests. I had lost 4.2 pounds, weighing in at 199 pounds, and although that was better, my doctor said that according to the recent labs I had taken, it appeared that I was a type 2 diabetic. I thought I was hearing things, the palms of my hands got sweaty, and I didn't know what to think. I was numb and in disbelief; you could have heard a pin drop. Then my doctor said that I would need to start on Metformin to help lower my A1C. She had my prescription called in. I picked it up, but I decided not to take it until I did some research on what type of drug Metformin was and its side effects. Also, I researched information on A1C and what I could do to lower it naturally, without prescription drugs. That day, I made up my mind that I needed to desperately try a lifestyle change, and taking medication for diabetes was not an option for me and certainly not for the rest of my life—no way! When I got home that day from my doctor's office, I went into my pantry and threw out all the GMO products: white flour, white sugar, white rice, pastas, chips, etc. My focus now was on eating a plant-based food diet and changing to a low-carb, low-sugar, high protein diet. I had a strong unction that this plan would bring me the results I needed to come off of medication and live a healthier, longer life. I met with Dr. Tassie, my holistic wellness doctor and after sharing my lab results with her, she put me on a basic clean diet and gave me a glycemic index chart, which is used to measure how much blood sugar stress a type of food creates, and also a daily journal to record and track my eating habits. I met with her weekly and began to work three or more days per week with a trainer at the Planet Fitness, and that was the start of my journey to better health. After a couple of months, I began to eat the foods listed under the anti-inflammatory Mediterranean diet in *Let Food Be Your Medicine* by Dr. Don Colbert. Through Dr. Colbert's book, I discovered how certain foods can heal the body and learned that I needed to make some serious dietary changes in order to reverse diabetes and lower my blood pressure, A1C, and cholesterol. Well, long story short, I tried it, and it worked. As it turned out, my healing remedy was food and exercise, and from that day on I began to look at food as my medicine. As I began the journey to following my new lifestyle change, within a week, I started to feel better. Day by day and week by week I received results that proved that with right diet, nutrition and exercise you can reverse such diseases as high blood pressure, high cholesterol and type 2 diabetes.

Please Read: Very Important

I am not a doctor; this book is based on my experience, results and research. My health was on a decline, and in less than four months it was completely turned around. I no longer have high blood pressure, diabetes, high cholesterol, high A1C, and etc. Nothing in this book is intended to treat you. Do not stop use of your medication. Please seek your doctor's advice before making any decisions that could affect your health, particularly if you suffer from any medical conditions or have symptoms that may require treatment.

2. **First Step – Your Why**

Develop a strong "Why." The reason why you want to make this new lifestyle change. It's sometimes hard to admit, but we can all sometimes face food temptations along the way and your "why" will be a strong reference source in helping you to get back on course.

Important Things to Do

Empty your pantry and home of all unhealthy foods.

Shop for healthy foods like fruits and green vegetables, particularly high-fiber foods and plant-based foods.

Read nutritional fact labels on all foods and beverages before purchasing.

Plan meals purposefully; watch portion sizes when eating meats and carbs.

Be sure your diet is low carb, low sugar, and high protein.

Keep a journal of the food you eat and exercise you do daily.

Be sure to eat five meals per day (breakfast, snack, lunch, snack, dinner).

Prep your fresh fruits and vegetables and put them in storage containers; this makes it so much easier to plan your meals, put your meals together, and saves you a lot of time and effort.

Read magazines, books, and various information on healthy foods daily.

Get involved with a nutritional support group.

See or follow a nutritionist, holistic, or naturopathy doctor on line, TV, or buy their books.

Keep measuring cups and measuring spoons on hand.

Exercise three or more times per week, daily if possible.

For exercise, purchase a resistance band loop, this helps when you are not able to go out and exercise, or for those who are unable to stand and exercise because of their conditions.

Know Your Food Enemies

Following is a list of foods and beverages I eliminated from my diet right away. They are enemies to your body and will inhibit you from maintaining optimal health. But before that, I have a word of caution for you.

My advice for you: **Keep them out!** These foods can cause harm and, if eaten too often, can cause mass destruction to your body, such as high cholesterol, high blood sugar levels, cancer, sugar diabetes, etc. So unless you can maintain control of how often you eat these foods, I sincerely recommend that you eliminate them. It gets tempting once you begin to eat them, especially sweets, as sugar is addictive. If you eat a bite of pizza, the taste of all that cheese and bread is so inviting, it's almost as though it's wooing you in, or calling your name. Donuts, hot cornbread…man, they're so delicious, tempting, and can breed obesity in the long or short run. It depends on a lot of factors, as everyone's circumstances are not equal. I have even noticed that some restaurant cooks are adding sugar to some of the foods that do not require sugar, like vegetables. You must watch out for sugar. I believe it's being added to keep you coming back. You wonder why we have such a problem with obesity, diabetes, and certain other diseases. I believe we definitely have a sugar problem.

To achieve your health goals and for quicker results I recommend that you eliminate the foods that are listed altogether as I did, particularly for the first four to six months, as this is when you have to work the hardest to implement new and good nutritional lifestyle changes to get your health back on track.

Foods you should eliminate from your diet:

Refined and processed foods	Pasta
White flour	Cheese
White sugar	Red meat
White bread (all bread)	Fried foods
White rice	Animal fat

Cakes, cookies, donuts, pastries, pies, ice cream, energy drinks, sodas, sweet tea, sweet breakfast cereals, biscuits, cornbread, French fries, beef, pork, sausage, ham, bacon, lunch meat, corn, microwave or ready meals, fast food, chips and genetically modified foods also known as (GMO'S). We must understand that the foods we eat can either heal or destroy our bodies. When eaten, some of the foods listed above can turn into sugar in your body. It's time to take a deep look at what we are eating. If the food we are eating isn't live foods, they are dead foods. Live foods are foods that have not been heated to the point at which the enzymes are destroyed. Live foods are raw foods, which include fruits, vegetables, seeds, nuts, sprouts, grains, sprouted legumes, spirulina, chlorella, and fruit juices (without artificial sweeteners). Live foods are foods that grow in the dirt and on trees; they occur naturally in nature. Dead foods are foods that can sit on your counter for days or weeks and not go bad. They are processed or highly processed refined foods, and most times they are synthetic and have very little or no nutritional value. As I was writing this book, a dear friend of mine who gave me permission to use her name, Monica, said that she could not give up her bacon. I sincerely pray that if you feel the same way, that the following research will change your mind.

I found out in my research that African Americans eat more bacon, ham, sausage, and other prepared meats than other groups. These foods have carcinogens, which are anything that lacks oxygen. Carcinogens are substances that are capable of causing cancer in living tissue. Within the Afro-American population, pancreatic cancer is 50 percent more frequent, and colon cancer is 20 percent more frequent, Now, I know that this is a real eye opener for many of us. (Encyclopedia of Foods and Their Healing Power 2001)

3. Choosing Foods That Give Life – Vegetables & Fruits

The Best food choices are fruits and vegetables because they are from nature, created by God. *Genesis 1:29,* KJV says, *"And God said, 'Behold I have given you every herb bearing seed, which is upon the face of all the earth, and every tree, in the which is the fruit of a tree yielding seed; to you it shall be for meat.'"* You can read this verse in the (AMP) that says, *"Every tree with seed in its fruit. You shall have them for food."* I believe God was saying that this food was to be our main course, because God said that this will be your food in the Bible. I know now, for myself, how healthy fruits and vegetables are for optimal health. I believe it was what turned my health around.

According to *USDA* many people need to eat 2 cups from the fruits group each day and 2 ½ cups from the vegetables group each day, see (*Vegetables and Fruits-Simple Solutions 2014).* The amounts noted above are for a person on a 2,000-calorie daily food plan. The amount of fruits and vegetables may vary depending on age, gender, physical activity, and overall health. I practiced this recommendation and am a witness to how much of a difference my health has improved as a result of eating more fruits and vegetables daily. The benefits of vegetables are low sodium, low fat, low calories, rich fiber, rich sources of iron, magnesium, calcium, vitamin C, and zero cholesterol. I recommend eating green vegetables at every meal. Green vegetables are like medicine—a natural pharmacy of minerals, vitamins, and phytochemicals. It is so important that we consume the proper number of servings of vegetables and fruits per day. When cooking vegetables, use very little water, if it's needed, and be careful not to overcook, because most vegetables have water in them.

Oxygen - Rich Foods

Foods that are rich in oxygen can improve your overall health; these are the foods that are most important to eat. When there is a lack of oxygen in the cells of the body, those deprived cells can become prime locations for cancer and other diseases. The way you receive the most oxygen from your food is by eating mostly raw green vegetables, as well as fruits, nuts, and sprouted seeds. Green vegetables contain chlorophyll. When you eat green vegetables, the chlorophyll allows blood to transport oxygen to cells.

(www.howtooxygenateyourbody2014). Green leafy vegetables are very high in chlorophyll. The two highest in chlorophyll are spinach and parsley. Other leafy greens are:

Collards Seaweed
Watercress Green tops of beets and turnips
Romaine lettuce
Arugula
Spirulina
Kelp

Processed and highly processed foods are unhealthy for the body, and a healthy diet is crucial. In my research, I have learned that an acidic diet can lead to breathing problems, cardiovascular disease, and other various, terminal diseases. (www. howtooxygenateyourbody2014)

A list of oxygen-rich foods with a high pH that should be in your diet are: Avocados, berries, carrots, celery, garlic, dates, apples, grapes, pears, raisins, pineapple, watercress, peppers, melons, grains, legumes, asparagus, parsley, papaya, limes, lemons, spinach, bell peppers, green beans, alfalfa sprouts, apricots, ripe bananas, etc.

Low Glycemic Vegetables

When I was diagnosed with diabetes, high cholesterol, and high A1Cs, Dr. Tassie, my Holistic Wellness doctor, put me on a basic clean diet. She gave me a glycemic food chart and expressed to me the importance of eating the foods that were low glycemic. The fruits that were safer to eat and that would keep my blood sugar under control were that from the berry family, such as; strawberries, raspberries, blackberries and etc. I suggest that you download a glycemic index chart for fruits and vegetables, as there are numerous types of charts and nutritional information on the internet to keep as a handy guide. It's also good to know what's in the foods you are eating when eating out. Ask questions about the foods you are ordering, as I often do. After all, we are not the cook, so that makes us unsure of what type of oils, seasonings, and other products they are using in the foods they are preparing for us to eat. If you need the cook to hold a seasoning, ask him or her to do so. Remember, what you eat can affect your health and how you function physically, emotionally, and psychologically.

Listed below are vegetables with a low glycemic index that are safe for people with diabetes because they avoid sugar spikes and they are:

Broccoli	Garlic
Collard Greens (and other green leafy veg's)	Turnips Beets
Cauliflower	Tomatoes
Squash	Zucchini
Sweet potatoes	Peas
Bell peppers (all colors)	Bok Choy
Green Salad (all kinds… arugula, romaine)	Kale Cabbage
Onion	Cucumbers
Radishes	Brussel Sprouts
Asparagus	Artichoke

Healthy Fruits to Eat

Fruit is the best and most natural source of vitamins, minerals, and fiber, and thus the most healthful. One can live without certain foods, but without fresh fruits and vegetables, it is impossible to remain healthy. The human body's overwhelming need for vitamin C can only be naturally met by eating fresh fruits. Although some vegetables also contain vitamin C, the primary dietary source of vitamin C is fruit. See the oxygen-rich

11

fruits listed under oxygen-rich foods located on the previous page. Fruit should be a part of your everyday diet. People who eat more fruit and vegetables as part of an overall healthy diet are likely to have a reduced risk of some chronic diseases (Nutrients and Health Benefits, 2015). To maintain a healthy body, one should include fruit as a part of his or her daily diet because it is an important source of many nutrients, such as fiber, vitamin C, and potassium. Fruit is a synonym of good health. No other type of food has so many preventive and healing properties as recorded in the (Encyclopedia of Foods and Their Healing Power 2001). Some nutrition specialists see each piece of fruit as a true natural medication. I remember the old saying, "An apple a day will keep the doctor away."

Here's a List of Some Healthy Fruits to Eat:

Avocados	Oranges Lemons
Tomatoes	Apples Watermelon
Blackberries	Pears Cherries
Strawberries	Grapefruit Guava
Raspberries	Pomegranate
Blueberries	Mango
Peaches	Cranberries

Plant-Based Nutritional Supplements:

Because life can sometimes be very busy, I found another way to get the daily recommended amount of fruits and vegetables, and it's by taking plant-based nutritional supplements. I keep on hand in my pantry also various concentrated superfood greens, "nutritional powerhouses" that supply my body with Phytonutrients (antioxidants), which are key to a healthy diet. I take them when I am on the go. I like to prepare them in my shaker cup, so I can easily drink my greens as I am driving in my car.

Choice of Nutritional Supplements That I Use:

Proteins and greens dietary supplements

Raw organic meal shake & meal replacement

Green Joy stackable salad bar superfoods (cacao and greens)

Juice Plus±, a blended fruit and vegetable juice powder in a capsule

Organic juice cleanse

Wheat grass

Spirulina

Greens concentrated superfood

4. **Meats and Other Healthy Food Sources**

During the recovery of my health I ate 3-5 ounces of meat up to twice per day, three to five days per week. Those meats are listed below:

Chicken (roasted, baked, grilled, blackened; skinless and **not fried**)

Tuna (if canned, choose one in water, not oil)

Salmon (fresh, wild caught, preferably pink in color)

Turkey (extra lean and ground)

I will however occasionally eat other types of seafood such as sardines, mackerel, herring, oysters and lake trout.

Other Healthy Foods

Beans and legumes: black beans and various other beans: chickpeas, lentils, split peas (good sources of fiber and protein)

Nuts: almonds, walnuts, cashews, macadamias

Seeds: sesame, pumpkin, flax, chia

Almond butter

Oils: extra virgin olive and avocado are both good sources of monounsaturated fat

Lite vinaigrette dressings

Hummus

Rice: brown rice only; I recommend brown rice because it is a whole grain and research shows that it's also less likely to raise your blood sugar than white grains. All brown rice is unrefined, better for your blood sugar, and will not cause blood sugar spikes when eaten moderately.

Types of Sugars and Sweeteners I Use

Lakanto Monk Fruit Sweetener 1:1: Is a non-gmo, zero-calorie, zero-glycemic sweetener that tastes and looks like white sugar. It is suitable for diabetics and is a natural product extracted from a dried fruit called monk fruit. The combination of this sweetener is monk fruit extract and non-gmo erythritol. For more information go online to: (https://www.lakanto.com)

Coconut Sugar: Coconut sugar is a palm sugar produced from the sap of the flower bud stem of the coconut palm. It is a natural sweetener that yields some tremendous benefits that make it a much better choice than many other sweetener options. Coconut sugar is better for diabetics and the gut than your normal, everyday sugar, and it holds trace amounts of vitamins and minerals. I personally have found coconut sugar to have a much better effect on my blood sugar levels than white sugar. However it is very important to remember that eating too much sugar, in any form, is not a good idea. (https://www.draxe.com)

One day my mother shared with me, how she noticed that when she used white sugar, she would experience an unusual feeling in her body. I suggested that she try coconut sugar. After using it, she noticed that she no longer felt that unusual feeling she did when she used white sugar. I have found zero problems after using coconut sugar, and as I stated before, it is a low-glycemic product.

My Choice of Beverages

Water is the most important and much needed drink that we can have. As a matter of fact, we cannot live without water. Water flushes our kidneys and is essential for other bodily functions. Water also helps with weight loss, whereas sugary drinks, such as sodas, energy drinks, sports beverages, and some fruit juices, are high in calories and caffeine. These can raise your blood pressure, your weight, and blood sugar, and should be avoided. Calcium from animal milk is not absorbed as well as that from plant-based sources so I made a switch long ago to a milk with lower calories and zero saturated fat. It's listed below along with the other beverages that I drink.

Almond Milk

Water

Lemon water

Coconut water

PowerAde (zero sugar) occasionally after physical workouts

Herbal teas and decaf coffee (occasionally)

Pedialyte (to hydrate and replace electrolytes)

5. **My Amazing Results and Lab Work**

Results:

Lost 48lbs pounds in four months

No more diabetes

Did not go on Metformin, as prescribed by my doctor

Lowered my A1C to the normal range

High blood pressure reversed

Came off of my high blood pressure medication after thirteen years

No more pain or stiffness in my joints

No more swollen ankles

Increased level of energy

Able to run upstairs two at a time

Went from a size 16 women's to a size 10 misses

Lowered my total cholesterol, lowered my LDL, and increased my HDL

I feel twenty-five years old again.

My Lab Results

Listed below are the lab results of my medical records from the start of my diagnosis, of type 2 diabetes in September 2016 to January 2017. I included them to show my progress along the way and to provide proof that if you follow the lifestyle plan in this book, you too can receive excellent results.

My First Visit

Date of Visit: 9/21/2016

Reason for Visit: Annual Wellness CPX/Patient has form for Dr. to sign/Needs fasting labs

Vitals:

Weight 203 (lbs.)

Height 66 (in.)

BP 146/84

BMI 32.83 (Index)

Medication List:

Lisinopril: 20 mg, 1 tablet every day, 30 days, refills: 1

Date of Visit: 9/28/2016

Reason for Visit: Discuss diabetes

Vitals:

Weight 199.2 (lbs.)

Height 66 (in.)

BP 151/82

BMI 32.15

Medication List:

Start Metformin HCI: 500 mg, 1 tablet with meals daily, 30 day(s), 30 tablets, refills: 2 Other medications you are on: Lisinopril: 20 mg, 1 tablet every day, 30 days, refills: 1

Date of Visit: 12/12/2016

Reason for Visit: Sinus and blood pressure check

Medication List:

Stop Lisinopril: 20 mg, 1 tablet every day, 30 days, refills: 1

Stop Metformin HCl: 500 mg, 1 tablet with meals daily, 30 day(s), 30 tablets, refills: 2

Start Lisinopril: 10 mg, as directed daily, 30 days, 30 tablets, refills: 11 (tablet decreased to half because of lower blood pressure, due to weight loss)

Date of Visit: 01/13/2017

Reason for Visit: Discuss blood pressure since weight loss

Lab: AlC – 5.0

Vitals:

Weight: 167.4 (lbs.)

HT: 65 (in)

BP: 120/79

BMI: 27.85

HR 70 (/min)

Other medications you are on:

Lisinopril: 10 mg, as directed daily, 30 days, 30 tablets, refills: 1

Discontinued Lisinopril: 20 mg, 1 tablet every day

Medication List:

None

Discontinued Lisinopril: 10 mg

Lab Results

September 21, 2016:

Triglycerides – 93

HDL - 48.0

LDL – 138

Total Cholesterol – 205

HbA1C – 6.6

November 17, 2016:

Triglycerides – 81

HDL – 35

LDL – 142

Total Cholesterol – 193

HbA1C – 5.7

Date of Visit: Jan 13, 2017

No more medicine; stop medications HBP/ Metformin per my doctor.

HbA1C – 5.0

6. Make the Right Choice for Better Health

- Swap GMOs and processed foods for plant-based foods.

- Eat plenty of fresh fruits and vegetables daily.

- Eat foods low in sugar and carbs and high in protein and fiber.

- Choose foods that are low in saturated fat.

- Eat foods that heal the body.

- Exercise three or more days per week for at least thirty minutes.

- Watch your portion and serving sizes.

- Use a food scale to measure and weigh your foods.

- Prep your food portions ahead each day to avoid overeating.

- Maintain a food journal (until you learn better eating habits).

- Read nutritional labels on all foods and beverages.

- Check the glycemic index chart for the amount of sugar, sodium, saturated fat, etc., in the fruits and vegetables you choose to eat. Remember, you are what you eat!

- Eat for good health and long living.

- God created our bodies, and we must remember that what we put into our bodies is by our choice. Choosing to eat healthy foods is choosing life.

- Use a food journal as a guide to record what you are eating.

- Keep in mind your "Why." If you fall off the wagon, your "why" can help you get on track again.

Important: To avoid drops in your blood sugar, try not to skip meals. If possible, a good recommendation would be to eat five small meals per day, including breakfast, lunch, dinner, and two snacks, as I do every two to three hours, because it's better for your metabolic rate.

7. **My Passion to Help Others**

I am living proof that diet and exercise, these two healthy lifestyle choices do work because they have made a significant change in my health and quality of life. I have learned that taking pharmaceutical drugs can help in a lot of cases however it does not always cure, as it did not cure my blood pressure. But healthy lifestyle choices brought better results and reversed the disease for which I was being treated for, for over thirteen long years. As I was writing this book, I received a call from a dear friend who needed my advice because she was having problems controlling her food cravings. I asked her what were the foods that she was craving, and she said that they were sweets, such as cookies, cake, and candy. She also craved chips. As I began to think of some food substitutes to suggest to her, I received a revelation that unhealthy foods are like enemies on a battlefield. So I thought, "*Hmm, yes that makes absolute sense.*" When we eat healthy foods, we are protecting our bodies from harm. When we choose to eat unhealthy foods, "the enemies" to our health, which are processed foods, gmo's, white sugar, white flour, etc., they will invade and eventually destroy our bodies and for some of us our lives, if we do not guard ourselves by making the right lifestyle choices. It's been said that "we are what we eat." I devote my time in studying and learning more about good nutrition and how it heals the body.

My Purpose and How I Discovered It

Growing up as the middle child in my family, I remember times when my three younger siblings would become ill with either a cold, flu, upset stomach or something of that nature. I being the oldest of the three, would find myself many times looking for something I could give to help them feel better. So when there was no medicine in the medicine cabinet, I would mix a few things together from the kitchen, stir it in a cup, give it to them and say, "here drink this," it will make you feel better.

Also, a couple of months before my dad went home to be with the Lord, I had a strong feeling inside that I needed to go and spend a week with him. Every year for my birthday my husband and I take a vacation to my place of choice. That particular year, as I so stated, I sensed God telling me to go home to spend time with my father and that I was to take care of him for the entire week of my stay. I didn't know it would be my last time with my dad. But God did, and I believe He allowed me the time to be with and care for my dad because He knew how much I loved him and he gave me the desire of my heart. When I was a young girl, I told my dad I would never leave him and that I would take care of him forever. Yes, I was a daddy's girl.

It was Monday morning, I arrived to my dad's house early before my stepmother left for work. She began to show me how to check my father's blood sugar and blood pressure. My father had both diabetes and heart trouble. So for that entire week, after she left for work, it was just Dad and I home every day. One day, I went to the grocery store and bought vegetables to make a pot of homemade soup. My dad ate the soup, but it did not have much seasoning. It lacked the taste that he desired and was use to eating. He loved eating breakfast from McDonald's, cakes, lemon pies and so much more. But I made sure that for one week, from morning to evening before I left for the day, he ate the right foods.

I can clearly see when I look back over all the years of my life, the many times I've spent encouraging people to eat healthy, that it was God bit by bit revealing His purpose for my life. Once I was offered a free course in food, nutrition, and health from the University of Georgia. It was during a time when my grandchildren were younger and their parents were working, that I met with a lady for several months who taught me a one-on-one course called, "Eating Right Is Basic." She was an extension nutrition program assistant, trained and supervised by county extension family and consumer science agents. I learned how to make healthy food choices and how to prepare healthy meals for my family.

In 2014, two years after undergoing six surgeries and one year of chemotherapy drugs for the treatment of breast cancer, I found myself again receiving a call from a representative who worked with a home health educational company that wanted to drop by our home on short notice, as she was visiting our area. I cannot remember what my reply was, but she came by, spent a couple of hours with me, and introduced me to some awesome health books: an education and health library that consisted of encyclopedias of fruits and vegetables and how they heal your body, medicinal plants and herbs, and healthy recipes. I was so impressed with the material that I decided to purchase the entire library of books.

Today, I pursue my interest and studies as a nutrition and wellness consultant. My passion and goal is to educate and enlighten people on how to take charge of their health. I serve as a volunteer in one of the local Hospital departments that care for cancer patients. I started a healing school ministry, which is for the purposes of educating, giving support, and empowering people in nutrition and healthy lifestyle choices.

8. Sample Meal Food Journal (Blank Copy) You Can Use as a guide

Week of: _____

	SUN	MON	TUES	WED	THURS	FRI	SAT
Breakfast							
Snack							
Lunch							
Snack							
Dinner							
Hydrate							

My Sample Meal Journal

Week of:_____

	SUN	MON	TUE	WED
Breakfast	**10 oz. Raw Meal Protein Shake**	**1 cup Homemade stew with 3 oz. chicken ½ cup black beans ½ cup mixed veggies**	**1/2 Avocado, 2 tomato slice 3 oz. ground turkey**	**3 oz. Ground turkey 1 avocado 5 grilled asparagus spears**
Snack	**10 Almonds 1/2 pear**	**10 Almonds**	**4-5 Ricecrackers w/ nut butter**	**1/2 apple, 3 crackers with nut butter**
Lunch	**1 Chicken thigh 1 cup Green beans 2 Lettuce Leaves 2 Tomato slices**	**4oz Salmon 1 cup Broccoli ½ cup Black beans**	**3 cups Veggie Salad, w/ squash, kale, bell peppers**	**10 inch plate Mixed salad with Kale Squash Bell peppers Black olives**
Snack	**3-5 Whole grain crackers**	**1/2 Apple**	**½ cup Raspberries**	**10 Almonds**
Dinner	**2 ½ cups Grilled chicken salad**	**3 oz. Ground turkey, 1 cup stewed veggies**	**2 cups Chicken soup w/ veggies**	**4 oz. Salmon 5 grilled Asparagus spears with spring mix salad**
Snack Optional	**NONE**	**½ Apple**	**NONE**	**½ Avocado**

	THUR	FRI	SAT
Breakfast	3 oz. Ground turkey, 8 oz. Raw Meal Protein Shake	1 egg white, 2 strips turkey bacon	1 boiled egg 1/3 cup of raisin bran with skim milk
Snack	5-6 almonds	8 almonds 5 wholegrain crackers	10 walnuts
Lunch	2 cup Vegetable Soup with Chicken, & Lentils	4 oz. grilled chicken breast salad with vinaigrette dressing	Greek salad with grilled chicken, Greek dressing
Snack	6 Strawberries	1 cup cauliflower, 1 stalk celery, red bell pepper	5 whole grain crackers 2 Tbsp. almond butter
Dinner	4 oz. Salmon, 1 cup green beans ½ sweet potato	3 oz. grilled chicken breast, 1 cup broccoli, ½ cup brown rice	3 oz. pan-seared tuna, 2 cup spinach, veg. cabob
Snack Optional	NONE	2/3rd cup Blackberries	1/2 energy bar

Hydrate: My recommendations are that you hydrate as often throughout the day as possible. Drink plenty of water and unsweetened beverages.

Portion Sizes

Always remember to keep your serving size. You can use a measuring cup or buy the portion size cups. I've learned that when trying to lose weight, it is very important that you watch your portion sizes. Eating five small meals per day will bring great results in your weight, metabolic rate, and overall health. If you increase your portion size of healthy foods, please be aware that you will still need to exercise to keep from gaining unwanted pounds over time. I've recently experienced this myself, so the solution I have come up with is to, again, start logging what you eat and drink throughout the day and stay consistent with exercising, even if it means getting down on the floor and doing some sit-ups at the end of the day. Because many of us have busy lives, it's easy to fall into the routine of eating out, so it's important not to over-eat at buffet-style restaurants or restaurants that are a la carte and serve large portions of foods. I found the best thing to do is ask for a carry-out container in which to take your food home; that way, you can eat it for another meal. Keep in mind that large portions of meat and carbs can easily cause the inches and pounds that you've taken off to sneak back up on you, especially if you do not exercise. Calories in will stay in, if you do not exercise. Just as a rule of thumb, remember that your plate should look something like this one below:

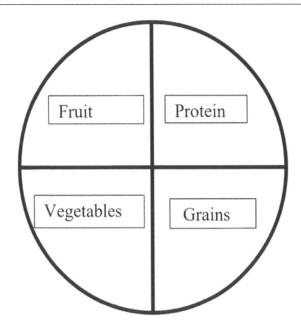

Make this eating style an everyday choice, as everything you eat and drink matters. You can find diagrams such as this by going online to www.choosemyplate.gov. Make half of your plate fruits and vegetables (eat plenty of fruits of all colors and a variety of vegetables). If you are not able to eat fruit at every meal, try doubling up on your vegetables, making at least half your plate vegetables. Eat various whole grains, like whole grain pasta, brown rice, and whole grain bread (if you desire bread). Choose a variety of protein such as: beans, nuts, fish, and poultry. According to USDA.ChooseMyPlate. gov the amount of fruits and vegetables you need to eat depends on age, sex, and level of physical activity. I believe that having a healthy body starts with a healthy plate.

9. Nutritional Terms and Definitions [1-25]

1. **Refined and processed carbohydrates**: Refined and processed carbohydrates are products made with white bleached flour and white rice which can cause insulin levels to spike. They get absorbed quickly in our system and raises our blood sugar level, and strips away beneficial fiber.

2. **Refined Sugar**: Refined sugar comes from sugar cane or sugar beets, which are processed to extract the sugar. It is typically found as sucrose, which is the combination of glucose and fructose. We use white and brown sugars to sweeten cakes and cookies, coffee, cereal, and other foods. Consuming too much refined sugar can promote and increase inflammation, and lead to weight gain. It can also raise your risk of diabetes and other chronic problems.

3. **Whole Grain**: Whole grains are grains of any cereal and pseudo-cereal that contain the endosperm, germ, and bran, in contrast to refined grains, which retain only the endosperm. Examples of whole grains include millet, spelt, brown rice, buckwheat, rye, and oats, and they are all high in fiber, contain more minerals, and are less processed than refined grains.

4. **Fiber**: Fiber is often known as roughage. It is the structural part of plants that the body cannot digest or absorb. Fiber is important in keeping your intestinal tract healthy and strong. It has been associated with helping to lower blood glucose levels and blood cholesterol levels, as well as the risk of colon cancer and cardiovascular disease. It also helps to relieve constipation.

5. **Nutrition Facts or Supplement Facts**: Nutrition facts or supplement facts are labels that reveal what's in the foods we eat and beverages we drink. You can find them on most packaged or processed products. Even though these labels are sometimes overlooked, it is very important to check your nutrition facts to know what you are eating, and don't forget the ingredient list. These two features are very important because you would not want to double your calories, sodium, carbohydrates, sugar, or other nutrients, which could be very harmful to your body. Below is a sample chart and a list of nutrition facts with their meanings. It is extremely important to read the nutrition facts on all your labels.

Nutrition Facts

Serving Size 1 cup (228g)
Servings Per Container about 2

Amount Per Serving

Calories 250   Calories from Fat 110

	% Daily Value*
Total Fat 12g	18%
Saturated Fat 3g	15%
Trans Fat 3g	
Cholesterol 30mg	10%
Sodium 470mg	20%
Total Carbohydrate 31g	10%
Dietary Fiber 0g	0%
Sugars 5g	
Proteins 5g	

Vitamin A			4%
Vitamin C			2%
Calcium			20%
Iron			4%

* Percent Daily Values are based on a 2,000 calorie diet. Your Daily Values may be higher or lower depending on your calorie needs.

	Calories	2,000	2,500
Total Fat	Less than	65g	80g
Saturated Fat	Less than	20g	25g
Cholesterol	Less than	300mg	300mg
Sodium	Less than	2,400mg	2,400mg
Total Carbohydrate		300g	375g
Dietary Fiber		25g	30g

For educational purposes only. This label does not meet the labeling requirements described in 21 CFR 101.9.

The example of the above nutrition fact and how to read a nutrition facts label can be found online at: familydoctor-org.cdn.ampproject.org.

Note: The serving size here is one cup. If you were to eat 2 cups, everything doubles, 3 cups it triples. For instance, with 2 cups, the calories would be 500, and if you do not burn those calories received with some type of exercise, you will store them, or, in other words, you will be wearing them. I am not sure what this food item is, but I know it is not something that I would recommend eating. The carbs and sodium per serving are very high. So always, always watch your labels. An example of what's listed on the nutrition facts label is below.

6. **Serving Size**: A serving size is the recommended portion of food to be eaten. It tells you how much of a food or liquid is in a serving.

7. **Calories**: A calorie is a unit that is used to measure energy. Our bodies need calories for energy, but eating too many calories and not burning enough of them off through activity can lead to weight gain.

8. **Total Fat**: The total fat is the sum of saturated and unsaturated fats in food.

9. **Cholesterol**: Cholesterol is a type of fat found in your blood. Your liver makes cholesterol for your body. You also get can get cholesterol from the foods you eat. Meat, fish, eggs, butter, cheese, and milk all have cholesterol in them.

10. **Carbohydrate**: Any of a large group of organic compounds occurring in foods and living tissues, including sugars, starch, and cellulose. They contain hydrogen and oxygen in the same ratio as water (2:1) and can typically be broken down to release energy in the animal body.

11. **Simple Carbohydrate**: Simple carbs (bad carbs) are quickly broken down by the body to be used as energy. They are found naturally in foods, such as fruits, milk, milk products, and processed and refined sugars, such as raw sugar, brown sugar, corn syrup and high fructose corn syrup, glucose, fructose, sucrose, fruit juice

concentrate, candy, soft drinks, and more. Simple carbs are bad because they can cause major swings in your blood sugar levels. They are low in fiber and quickly digestible.

12. **Complex Carbohydrate**: Complex carbs (good carbs) are made up of sugar molecules that are strung together in long, complex chains. They are the good carbs found in foods such as peas, beans, whole grains, and vegetables. Both simple and complex carbs are turned to glucose (blood sugar) in the body and used as energy.

13. **Dietary Fiber**: Dietary fiber is a type of carbohydrate that cannot be digested by our bodies' enzymes. It is found in edible plant foods, such as cereals, fruits, vegetables, nuts, dried peas, grains, and lentils. Fiber is grouped by its physical properties and is called soluble, insoluble, or resistant starch. Both soluble and insoluble fiber are important for digestion, health, and preventing disease. Soluble fiber attracts water and turns to gel during digestion. Insoluble fiber attracts water into your stool, making it softer and easier to pass with less strain on your bowel regulates bowel movements and prevents hemorrhoids. Insoluble fiber may reduce blood cholesterol and sugar, helping the body improve blood glucose control, which can aid in reducing your risk for diabetes. Resistant starch is any starch that is not digested in the small intestine but passes to the large bowel. Foods that are high in resistant starch are: oats, green bananas, beans, peas, lentils, cooked and

cooled rice, cooked and cooled potatoes, green beans, barley and raw potato starch.

14. **Sugar**: Sugar is a sweet, crystalline substance obtained from various plants, especially sugar cane and sugar beet, consisting essentially of sucrose and used as a sweetener in foods and drinks.

15. **Protein**: Protein is an essential nutrient for the human body. It is one of the building blocks of body tissue and can also serve as a fuel source.

16. **Vitamin**: A vitamin is an organic molecule, which is an essential micronutrient that an organism needs in small quantities to sustain life. Vitamins are substances that your body needs to grow and develop normally.

17. **Mineral**: A mineral is an inorganic element, such as calcium, iron, potassium, sodium, or zinc and it is essential to the nutrition of humans, animals, and plants.

18. **Saturated Fat**: Saturated fat is a type of fat that contributes to weight gain, heart disease, and diabetes. The American Heart Association recommends limiting saturated fats, which are found in butter, cheese, red meat, and other animal-based foods. Decades of sound science has proven it can raise your "bad" cholesterol, LDL, and put you at a higher risk for heart disease and stroke. (www.American Heart Association/fats/saturated.org).

19. **Monounsaturated Fat**: Monounsaturated fat is a healthy fat of an organic compound, especially a fat, saturated except for one multiple bond. Monounsaturated fat, for example olive oil, is thought to be healthier than saturated fat. Monounsaturated fats can be found in nuts, seeds, salmon, avocado, eggs, and seed oils, and are liquid at room temperature.

20. **Polyunsaturated Fat**: Polyunsaturated fat is a healthy fat that can be found in plant and animal foods, such as nuts, seeds, seed oils, fish, and oysters. Eating moderate amounts of polyunsaturated and monounsaturated fats, in place of saturated and trans fats, can benefit your health.

21. **Trans Fat**: Trans fats is another term for trans-fatty acid. Trans fats raise your bad (LDL) cholesterol levels and lower your good (HDL) cholesterol levels. Eating trans fats increase your risk of developing heart disease and stroke, and is associated with a higher risk of developing type 2 diabetes.

22. **Animal Fat**: Animal fat is lipid material derived from animals that is composed of triglycerides.

23. **Processed Foods**: Processed foods result from any deliberate change in a food that occurs before it is available for us to eat.

24. **GMO**: A genetically modified organism (GMO) is any organism whose genetic material or makeup has been altered using genetic engineering techniques.

25. **Sodium**: Salt is the term commonly used for sodium chloride (NaCl), which is table salt. Excess sodium increases blood pressure, because it holds excess fluid in the body, creating an added burden on the heart. Too much sodium will increase your risk of stroke, heart failure, kidney disease, osteoporosis, and stomach cancer.

10. Why I Chose Plant-Based Foods over Pharmaceutical Drugs

The reason I chose plant-based foods as my medicine over Metformin a pharmaceutical drug was the fear of harm that the prescription drugs side effects could cause to my body. Also, after receiving the diagnosis of diabetes from my physician and doing my own research on reversing diabetes the natural way, I thought I would have nothing to lose but everything to gain if I 'de give it a try. So I tried food as my medicine and have found it to have significant healing properties that have brought fantastic results. It not only reversed diabetes, but it lowered my A1C, LDL cholesterol, triglycerides, blood pressure, BMI, and weight. We have accepted that the only way to survive with an illness or disease is to be on pharmaceutical drugs for the rest of our lives. Now whereas that may be true for some, it is not true for all. The truth is some are not willing to work through the necessary changes to improve their health. It does take changing old habits, which can be a challenge. We can overcome food addictions, poor nutritional diets and lack of physical exercise, but it takes work.

Note: If you are on prescription drugs, do not stop the use without consulting with your doctor first. As your body begins to heal itself, and it will, your doctor will make the necessary changes in adjusting your prescription medications. All statements documented in this book are not intended to diagnose, treat, cure, or prevent disease, but are based on my own experiences, interest, and research on nutrition. As I so stated before, I am not a physician. Before trying any new diet or deciding to stop any of your medications, please talk with your doctor first.

What I Believe

In Genesis 1:29, the Bible records that God blessed the green plants and said they were good for us to eat. Even though we enjoy how other foods taste, because they taste good, it does not mean they are healthy or beneficial for us to eat. I do believe that some sicknesses and diseases have a lot to do with what we eat. The fact is when I changed my diet and began eating more plant-based foods, exercised three to five days per week, and dropped the excess weight, my health improved and diseases were reversed. God created heaven and earth. He made our bodies and told us what foods we should eat. Don't get me wrong: I used to enjoy barbeque ribs, fried chicken wings, corn bread, biscuits, macaroni 'n' cheese, cake, ice cream, sugary drinks, and other unhealthy, tasty, enjoyable foods too. But the truth is when we consistently eat unhealthy foods, it becomes a habit that is very hard to stop. Most times, as a result, we find ourselves overweight and obese, which opens the door for sickness and disease.

11. **Let Food Be Your Medicine**

Hippocrates was a Greek physician known as the "father" of Western medicine. One of his quotes was, "Let Food Be Thy Medicine and Medicine Be Thy Food." While I was writing this book, I realized that back in 2011, before I had received a diagnosis of cancer, I was not eating the recommended daily amount of fruits and vegetables and had a poorly balanced diet.

Listed below are some cancer-fighting foods and how they work according to (Karen Davis, Natures Healing Foods).

Apricot: Lowers the risk of cancer, especially smoking-related forms, such as lung cancer.

Asparagus: Packed with vitamins and minerals that help reduce the risk of cancer.

Barley: Has a combination of protective powers — manganese, molybdenum, and beta-glucans — nutrients that work together to prime your immune cells to aggressively seek out and destroy cancer cells. Consume 3 cups weekly.

Broccoli, Brussel Sprouts, and Cauliflower: Lower the risk of cancer, especially cancer of the stomach, colon, and lungs.

Cabbage: Lowers the risk of cancer, especially cancer of the colon.

Cantaloupe: Rich in nutrients, beta carotene, and vitamin C that may prevent cancer.

Carrots: Block cancer, especially smoking-related cancers.

Fig: Fights cancer.

Garlic: Contains cancer-preventive chemicals.

Garam Masala: A savory blend of ground spices used in Indian cuisine, which can energize the immune cells that fight cancer in two weeks. Consume ½ tsp. per day.

Grapefruit: Lowers the risk of cancer, especially cancer of the stomach and pancreas.

Legumes: Beans, peas, or lentils. Legumes are rich in fiber, which binds to toxins and excess hormones, zapping them out of the body before they contribute to cancer. Eat 1/2 cup daily

Lemon and Lime: Contain vitamin C that block cancer.

Milk: Inhibits certain cancers.

Onion: Blocks cancer.

Orange: Lowers the risk of some cancers.

Peas: Prevent cancer.

Spinach: Lowers the risk of cancer, especially lung cancer.

Squash and Pumpkin: Lower the risk of many kinds of cancer, especially lung cancer.

Strawberry: May prevent and lowers cancer-related deaths.

Sweet Potato: Lowers the risk of cancer.

Wheat Bran: Prevents colon cancer.

Tomato: Lowers risk of cancer.

Yogurt: Has anti-cancer ingredients

Foods That Heal and Helps to Reduce Your Cholesterol

Celery: Cleanses the blood and reduces cholesterol. Celery also acts as an alkalizer which eliminates acidic, metabolic residues. Celery has a diuretic effect and is particularly beneficial to those suffering from hypertension. A very important compound in celery is called apigenin, which is a potent anti-inflammatory that helps stall the growth and spread of even tough-to-treat cancers. It works by shutting down blood flow to cancer cells, starving them of the oxygen and nutrients they need to survive.

Walnuts: Walnuts are an excellent source of monounsaturated fats and omega-6 fats, and are great for heart health. These unsaturated fats help lower cholesterol levels, prevent blood clotting, and reduce the risk of sudden death from dangerous, abnormal heart rhythms.

Sesame Seeds: Of all the seeds and nuts, sesame seeds have the highest content of phytosterols, plant compounds that are believed to reduce blood cholesterol levels, boost your immune system, and reduce the risk of certain types of cancer. Sesame seeds are a good source of calcium. They also provide some relief from rheumatoid arthritis because of their high levels of copper, which has anti-inflammatory properties. Sesame seeds have magnesium that relaxes blood vessels and may benefit migraine-sufferers.

Fiber: Fiber is what gives strength and structure to plants. Most grains, vegetables, fruits, and beans contain fiber. A diet high in fiber helps your digestive system function better. Having a diet high in fiber can help you maintain a healthy weight. Fiber fills you up more, so you can eat less, and it reduces your risk for certain health problems, such as heart disease, diabetes, stroke, and some digestive diseases. Fiber helps to lower "bad" cholesterol in the blood. A healthy diet includes 14 grams of fiber for every 1,000 of the calories you eat each day. Choose whole foods that are naturally high in fiber. The closer a food is to nature, the less it is processed, and the better it is for you.

A List of High Fiber Foods:

Whole Grains – Brown rice, 100 percent whole grains

Fruits – Apples with skin on, oranges, pears, berries, bananas

Vegetables – Broccoli, greens, sweet potatoes, squash, asparagus, carrots, peas

Legumes – Lentils, dried beans, split peas, chickpeas

Nuts and Seeds – Almonds, sunflower seeds, chia seeds

Foods That Heal Your Pancreas and Liver:

It is very important to know that having a fatty liver may play a role in the development of type 2 diabetes. The pancreas produces insulin, which reduces blood sugar levels and allows your body to store food energy for future use. Eating the right foods can heal and nourish your pancreas.

Foods that heal the pancreas are garlic, lemons, blueberries, cherries, broccoli, spinach, cabbage, kale, leafy greens vegetables, sweet potatoes, carrots, squash, onions, Brussels sprouts, cauliflower, etc.

Whole Grains: Whole grains provide complex carbohydrates and B vitamins required for proper liver function.

Fruits: Apples, grapes, plums, cherries, loquat: These fruits promote the emptying of the bile and detoxify and relieve congestion of the liver. They also prevent constipation, provide antioxidants, are low in sodium and fats, are rich in vitamin A and minerals, and improve blood circulation.

Onions: Onions stimulate the detoxifying action of the liver because of their sulfureted, essential oil.

Lecithin: Lecithin contains choline, a vitamin factor that is essential to liver metabolism and to keep fat from depositing in the liver.

Olive Oil: Olive oil promotes liver health; take about 2-3 tablespoons daily.

Artichoke: Artichoke has a content called cynarin and other active substances. Cynarin improves liver function, detoxifies, and aids in the elimination of waste material with the bile.

Important: These statements have not been evaluated by the Food and Drug Administration. None of the products listed are intended to diagnose, treat, cure, or prevent any disease. This content is for informational and educational purposes only. It is not intended to provide medical advice or take the place of medical advice or treatment from a personal physician.

12. Teas and Herbs That Help in Healing

Green Tea: Green tea combats cancer and heart disease. Drinking green tea can lower blood sugar levels and help prevent type 2 (late onset) diabetes. It can also help prevent osteoporosis. Green tea can be used for treating diarrhea and for killing bacteria that is responsible for stomach upset. Green tea helps combat the flu virus also.

Black Tea: Black tea has antioxidant properties that may boost heart health. It may also help to reduce blood pressure, blood sugar levels, "bad" LDL cholesterol, the risks of stroke and cancer, and much more.

Hibiscus Tea: Hibiscus tea helps to lower LDL cholesterol and has antioxidants that help to support blood pressure. Hibiscus tea is rich in phytonutrients and is a good source of vitamin C.

Passion Flower Tea: Passion flower tea helps you to lose weight, and it aids in helping you to sleep and is effective in reducing anxiety.

Peppermint Tea: Peppermint tea supports digestive tract health and has anticancer, antioxidant, antiviral, and antibacterial properties. Peppermint tea is also used to relieve stomach pain and nausea.

Ginger Tea: Ginger tea is a healthy, disease-fighting antioxidant. It helps fight inflammation and stimulate the immune system, and is well known for its effectiveness in relieving nausea.

Echinacea Tea: Echinacea tea is a popular tea widely known for preventing and shortening the common cold. It may help boost the immune system, which could help the body fight off infections and viruses.

Lemon Balm Tea: Lemon balm tea has been found to improve the elasticity of the arteries, which lessens your changes of stroke, mental decline and heart disease. (Restivo Health and Wellness, 2019).

13. Exercise to Improve Your Health

Exercise is very essential for a long and healthy life, and very effective when combined with dieting to lose weight. I used to exercise occasionally, but meeting my trainer in 2016 changed my outlook on physical exercise forever. I truly believe God put him there in Planet Fitness just for me. He exhibited so much love and passion for exercise. He had a thorough way of teaching, and I could not have asked for a better trainer. He wasn't at the gym long, but long enough to give me the fundamentals, skills, and techniques of exercising. To start, the goal he set for me was twenty minutes of cardio and ten minutes of strength training. He then increased my length of time on the treadmill to thirty minutes and shortly after began to introduce me to the strength training equipment.

You will find that when you begin to lose weight and reach the right amount of weight loss, your energy will increase and your joints will stop aching. To me, exercise is now mandatory and should be a regular staple in our schedules. Exercise is not an option but a necessary lifestyle change that can help to keep your blood pressure under control. Strength training is helpful because muscle helps your body process glucose. Wow! You can build a sugar-proof body. I always say that I believe God made our bodies as "healing machines," and every machine has to be tuned up, worked, and kept moving in order for it to perform well. We need to begin to look further into the benefits of exercise, because I would say that most of us are probably not giving physical exercise the credit it deserves in our lives. Beginning to take exercise seriously is to our advantage. My perception has changed, and I now have respect for exercise where I did not before. Today, I have energy like I did when I was twenty years old. I sprint up the stairs two at a time. I am fifty-eight years young, not old. I feel great, really great. I can remember, before the weight loss, how difficult it was to even think about how I could get down and back up from the floor. I did not realize how physically unfit I had become. Once you are on the track of sliding down in your health, it becomes more difficult and challenging to come back up. Being overweight or obese can affect how you think too. I remember, before I lost the weight, if ever I needed to get down on the floor, I would say, "Forget it, I will not be able to get back up." Now, I'm sure I could have gotten up some way; however, I believe my weight had an effect on my thinking. Once I lost the weight, I noticed that I was able to get down on the floor, jump up on my feet, and sprint up the stairs two at a time without giving any thought as to how I would be able to do it. Combining eating right with exercise has lifelong benefits, and I feel it is important to keep a daily exercise log and food journal to assist you in being accountable for your health and wellness journey. Attached is an example of my daily exercise log, which you can use for yourself as a guideline.

My Sample Exercise Log

Month _____

	Sunday	Monday	Tuesday
Week of:_____	Treadmill-40 min. 1.60 miles 200 cal.	None	Treadmill-40.30 min. 2 miles 211 cal.
Week of:_____	Abs-15 min. Treadmill-35 min. 175 cal.	Treadmill-20 min. 100 cal. Strength	Treadmill-34 min. 120 cal. 1.40 miles
Week of:_____	None	Treadmill-30 min. 179 cal. Abs-30 min.	Treadmill-30 min. 144 cal. Strength-30 min.
Week of:_____	Treadmill-30 min. 174 cal.	None	Treadmill-30 min. 174 cal. Strength

	Wednesday	Thursday	Friday	Saturday
Week of:_____	None	Treadmill- 30 min. 140 cal.	Treadmill- 35 min. 175 cal. Abs- 5 min. Strength- 30 min.	None
Week of:_____	Treadmill- 30 min. 150 cal. Abs- 10 min.	Treadmill- 65 min. 316 cal. Abs- 2 min.	Crunches, Leg raises- 20 min. 123 cal.	None
Week of:_____	None	Treadmill- 30 min. 143 cal. Abs- 15 min.	Exercise bike- 20 min. Abs-15 min. 115 cal.	Treadmill- 30 min. 175 cal. Strength- 20 min.
Week of:_____	Treadmill- 40 min. 231 cal.	Treadmill- 30 min. 173 cal.	Strength Training - 20 min. 165 cal.	None

I want to add that while I was writing this book, I had the opportunity while shopping one day to come across a box of Therapy Loops, which are used for exercise. They are great to use while standing, sitting, or lying down, and you can use them on your arms or hands. They are made to stretch, so you are to pull on them; as you pull, you are able to feel the resistance. You can increase your resistance with light, medium, and strong loops.

I recommend these to everyone, especially those who find it difficult to exercise due to their inability to stand long, or those who are perhaps in a wheelchair. It's even great for senior citizens. You can find them online or in sporting goods stores and at Walmart.

14. **Healthy Recipe**:

Low-Sodium Salad Dressing

Recommended for those who are concerned about their blood pressure

Ingredients:

1/2 cup olive oil

2 tbsp. red vinegar

1 tsp. yellow mustard

1/2 tsp. minced garlic

A dab of paprika

I use this dressing for my salads, and
I recommend this dressing because it's low in sodium. The only amount of sodium in this dressing is 70 mg. per tsp., which is in the mustard. All the other ingredients have zero sodium.

Remember that store-bought dressings are high in sodium and should be used with caution! If you read the nutrition facts on the back of the bottle you will see that most times the milligrams (mg) per serving for dressings are 2 tablespoons (tbsp.), making it extremely necessary to measure out your servings. For instance, if the dressing is 430 mg of sodium per 2 tablespoons, then every additional time you fill that tablespoon, the amount of mg. goes up. This is where many of us go wrong. I've talked to quite a few people who say that they still have a problem with their blood pressure and do not know why. This is the area most times where they have not understood, or overlooked, that when you pour dressings over your salad without measuring it first, your milligrams of sodium intake can go up to the thousands.

15. The Word of God Is Our Medicine

Spiritual food is needed for spiritual growth. The Word of God is spiritual healing for our bodies. It is recorded in Matthew 4:4, "Jesus answered, 'It is written: Man shall not live on bread alone, but on every word that comes from the mouth of God.'"

Below are healing Scriptures to take by saying them with your mouth and believing them in your heart. Just as a doctor writes a prescription for you to take for a condition (diabetes, cholesterol, high blood pressure), it won't cure the disease or sickness, but you take it in hopes that it will keep you alive. For example, the prescription will read, "Take 1 tablet by mouth every morning," or, "Take 2 tablets by mouth twice daily." Well, likewise, I encourage you to take the Word of God as your medicine by speaking the following Scriptures daily as many times as you need for your situation or condition. "For life and death is in the power of your tongue, and those who love it will eat its fruit" (Prov. 18.21).

The following Scriptures are from the Holy Bible, taken from the NIV version.

Jeremiah 30:17:
"For I will restore health to you and I will heal your wounds; says the LORD."

Exodus 15:26:

"For I am the Lord, Who heals you."

Psalms 103:3:

"Who forgives all your sins and heals all your diseases."

3 John 1:2:

"Dear friend, I pray that you may enjoy good health and that all may go well with you, even as your soul is getting along well."

Proverbs 4:20-23:

"My son pay attention to what I say; turn your ear to my words. Do not let them out of your sight, keep them within your heart; for they are life to those who find them and health to one's whole body. Above all else, guard your heart, for everything you do flows from it."

Isaiah 53:4-5:

"Surely He took up our pain and bore our suffering, yet we considered Him punished by God, stricken by Him, and afflicted. But He was pierced for our transgressions, He was crushed for our iniquities; the punishment that brought us peace was on Him and by His wounds we are healed."

Deuteronomy 30:19:

"This day I call the heavens and the earth as witnesses against you that I have set before your life and death, blessings and curses. Now choose life, so that you and your children may live."

Psalm 118:17:

> "I will not die but live, and will proclaim what the Lord has done."

Mark 11:24:

> "Therefore I tell you, whatever you ask for in prayer, believe that you have received it, and it will be yours."

John 10:10:

> "The thief comes only to steal and kill and destroy; I have come that they may have life, and have it to the full."

1 Peter 2:24:

> "Who His own self bare our sins in His own body on the tree. That we, being dead to sins, should live unto righteousness: by whose stripes ye were healed."

Exodus 23:25:

> "You shall serve the Lord your God; He shall bless your bread and water, and I will take sickness from your midst."

Healthy Lifestyle Declarations

I will eat foods that bring healing to my body and quality of life.

I love life; I will live to see and have good day's ahead living in health and prosperity.

I can eat healthy, and I will do it day by day for a lifetime.

It is not God's will that I be sick.

I will take ownership of my health.

I love me.

I refuse to allow sickness to dominate my body.

The life of God flows within me, bringing healing to every fiber of my being.

I shall live and not die before my time.

God's purpose will be fulfilled in my life.

I will prosper and be in health, even as my soul prospers.

No weapon that is formed against me shall prosper.

I thank you, Heavenly Father, for my life is in Your hand.

Thank you Lord God that Your plan for my life is good and You're bringing me to an expected end.

I will live, I will live, and I will live all of my days in good health.

A Prayer of Blessing

Dear friend, I pray that you may enjoy good health and that all may go well with you, even as your soul is getting along well. May God bless you on your new journey of health and wellness, and I pray that my testimony and the information in this first volume blesses your life as it has blessed mine. I am looking forward to hearing that your health has turned around, and you're feeling more energized and healed of all sickness and disease. Peace to you, your home, and all that you have in Jesus's name.

Bibliography/Notes

1. Colbert, Don, MD. Let Food Be Your Medicine. 1st ed., Worthy Publishing Group, 2016, p. 39-53, "In Search of an Anti-Inflammatory Diet," and "The Anti-Inflammatory Diet"

2
First Step -Your Why

1. Pamplona-Roger, George D., MD. Encyclopedia of Foods and Their Healing Power. vol. 1, Review and Herald Publishing Association, 2001, p. 25

3
Choosing Foods That Give Life

1. https://www.snaped.fns.usda.gov/vegetables andfruits-simplesolutions/2014

2. Jain, Suneil. "How to Oxygenate Your Body." Rejuvenate Health & Aesthetics, accessed June 8, 2019, https://www.werejuvenate.com

3. Daiwik. "Top 10 Foods Rich In Oxygen." Stylecraze.com, accessed Oct 29, 2019, http://www.top10foodsrichinoxygen

4. "Nutrients and Health Benefits, Why Is It Important to Eat Vegetables." Choosemyplate.gov, USDA, accessed October 2, 2019, https://www.choosemyplate.gov/vegetables.

5. Pamplona-Roger, George D., MD. Encyclopedia of Foods and Their Healing Power. vol. 1, Review and Herald Publishing Association, 2001, p. 39

4

Meats and Other Healthy Food Choices

1. https://draxe.com/nutrition, "Is Coconut Sugar Good for You?" accessed Oct 30, 2019

2. Davis, Karen. Nature's Healing Foods. 1st ed., Globe Communications Corp., 1995, pp. 8, 14 96

3. Pamplona-Roger, George D., MD. Encyclopedia of Foods and Their Healing Power. vol. 2, Review and Herald Publishing Association, 2006, p. 249

Other Books by Cynthia Jones

My Sleep Shall "B" Sweet (2003), available by ordering online through Salem Authors, Amazon.com, Barnes and Noble, and all online Retailers.

If you would like to contact Cynthia Jones you can do so via:

Facebook.com/cynthiajones
Instagram: cynthia.jones
cynthiabjonesministries.com *(under construction)*